Hope and Help

A Planner for Cancer Patients Going Through
Chemotherapy Treatment

Bridgette Eilers

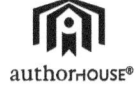

authorHOUSE®

AuthorHouse™
1663 Liberty Drive
Bloomington, IN 47403
www.authorhouse.com
Phone: 1-800-839-8640

First published by AuthorHouse   02/21/2012

ISBN: 978-1-4685-5399-4 (sc)
ISBN: 978-1-4685-5400-7 (hc)
ISBN: 978-1-4685-5401-4 (ebk)

Library of Congress Control Number: 2012903044

Printed in the United States of America

This Planner belongs to:

Name:		
Street Address:		
City:	**State:**	**Zipcode:**
Home Phone:		**Cell Phone:**
email:		

I hope that this planner helps you organize your chemotherapy journey.

Contents

Dedication

I dedicate this planner to my husband Gregg, my three amazing children, and my incredible family and friends who supported me and gave so willingly to me to make my chemo journey a success. Their efforts inspired me to put this planner together. I also want to thank God for guiding me through my chemotherapy journey and always being there for me when I thought I could not go on any longer. Without all of their love and support I would not be where I am today.

Introduction

My name is Bridgette Eilers. I was diagnosed with stage 3c Ovarian Cancer in March of 2011. When I heard the word cancer, I automatically thought, "Am I going to die? I am only 29. I have three young children. How could this be happening to me? This has got to be a mistake. Maybe the information got mixed up." I wanted so badly for the doctor to have made a mistake or misdiagnosed me. But the reality was, I had cancer. My husband and I left the doctors office in shock. We thought, "How are we going to tell our family, our friends, and our children? Our kids are so young, how are they going to understand?" Once my husband and I told our family, friends and our kids, we now had to think about the treatment plan. The plan was to surgically remove the cancer and then we would decide on how much, if any, chemotherapy was necessary. Well, after surgery, six rounds of chemotherapy was the plan. So from start to finish it would be six months of my life. It does not sound that long, but with three kids and a husband that worked full time, it felt like it would be a lifetime. "How am I going to do this? I can't be a mom, wife and chemotherapy patient." My chemo months were very difficult. I probably experienced 90% of the side effects that they tell you about.

That is where my amazing family and friends came in. My mom, sister, and in-laws traded weeks taking care of me. My dad, sister-in-law, and friends helped out with the kids. My friends took care of meals, house cleaning, and lawn care throughout my whole treatment. Their support helped me focus on getting better. They became my Chemo Crew.

Since treatment has finished I have had a passion and desire to help others who are going through chemotherapy treatment. I started The Chemo Crew, an organization that offers hope and help to anyone going through treatment. This planner was something I really could have used.

What I experienced during my journey was that there was a lot of medical advice, but there was not a lot of support and information from a survivor's perspective. So I hope these tips help you through your journey.

Remember, everyone is different, so do not believe everything that you read will happen to you. You are your own person and will respond in your own way. Try your best to prepare, but don't freak out if things don't go as planned. Instead of searching the Internet yourself, ask your doctor for some reliable websites that can give you the best and most up to date information.

Let people help you. If you are anything like me, you like to be in control. One of the hardest things for me was to let people help me. Communicate what you need and you will be amazed at the response. Remember that this is hard for them too, they want to help in any way possible.

Most importantly, remember you are not alone. There are way too many people who know what you are going through. Reach out and talk to other people who have been through treatment. There are many support groups out there.

I hope this planner gives you tips and ways to organize this time in your life. For more useful tips from a patients perspective visit my website at www.thechemocrew.com.

Contacts

Use this to write down important contacts. You will get a lot of phone numbers during this season in your life. You will receive many of business cards, flyers and info from doctors. If you have one place where you write them all, you will be able to easily locate them when you need them.

Important Contact Info:

Name:		
Street Address:		
City:	**State:**	**Zipcode:**
Home Phone:		**Cell Phone:**
email:		

Name:		
Street Address:		
City:	**State:**	**Zipcode:**
Home Phone:		**Cell Phone:**
email:		

Name:		
Street Address:		
City:	**State:**	**Zipcode:**
Home Phone:		**Cell Phone:**
email:		

Name:		
Street Address:		
City:	**State:**	**Zipcode:**
Home Phone:		**Cell Phone:**
email:		

Important Contact Info:

Name:	
Street Address:	
City: **State:**	**Zipcode:**
Home Phone:	**Cell Phone:**
email:	

Name:	
Street Address:	
City: **State:**	**Zipcode:**
Home Phone:	**Cell Phone:**
email:	

Name:	
Street Address:	
City: **State:**	**Zipcode:**
Home Phone:	**Cell Phone:**
email:	

Name:	
Street Address:	
City: **State:**	**Zipcode:**
Home Phone:	**Cell Phone:**
email:	

Important Contact Info:

Name:
Street Address:
City: State: Zipcode:
Home Phone: Cell Phone:
email:

Name:
Street Address:
City: State: Zipcode:
Home Phone: Cell Phone:
email:

Name:
Street Address:
City: State: Zipcode:
Home Phone: Cell Phone:
email:

Name:
Street Address:
City: State: Zipcode:
Home Phone: Cell Phone:
email:

Important Contact Info:

Name:		
Street Address:		
City:	**State:**	**Zipcode:**
Home Phone:		**Cell Phone:**
email:		

Name:		
Street Address:		
City:	**State:**	**Zipcode:**
Home Phone:		**Cell Phone:**
email:		

Name:		
Street Address:		
City:	**State:**	**Zipcode:**
Home Phone:		**Cell Phone:**
email:		

Name:		
Street Address:		
City:	**State:**	**Zipcode:**
Home Phone:		**Cell Phone:**
email:		

Important Contact Info:

Name:			
Street Address:			
City:	State:	Zipcode:	
Home Phone:		Cell Phone:	
email:			

Name:			
Street Address:			
City:	State:	Zipcode:	
Home Phone:		Cell Phone:	
email:			

Name:			
Street Address:			
City:	State:	Zipcode:	
Home Phone:		Cell Phone:	
email:			

Name:			
Street Address:			
City:	State:	Zipcode:	
Home Phone:		Cell Phone:	
email:			

Important Contact Info:

Name:		
Street Address:		
City:	**State:**	**Zipcode:**
Home Phone:		**Cell Phone:**
email:		

Name:		
Street Address:		
City:	**State:**	**Zipcode:**
Home Phone:		**Cell Phone:**
email:		

Name:		
Street Address:		
City:	**State:**	**Zipcode:**
Home Phone:		**Cell Phone:**
email:		

Name:		
Street Address:		
City:	**State:**	**Zipcode:**
Home Phone:		**Cell Phone:**
email:		

Medication Log

You will receive some new medications and may need to manage your existing prescriptions. Use this log to help keep yourself or your caregiver organized.

Medication Log

Prescription	Am	Pm	Am	Pm	Am	Pm	Am	Pm

Medication Log

Prescription	Am	Pm	Am	Pm	Am	Pm	Am	Pm

Medication Log

Prescription	Am	Pm	Am	Pm	Am	Pm	Am	Pm

Medication Log

Prescription	Am	Pm	Am	Pm	Am	Pm	Am	Pm

Medication Log

Prescription	Am	Pm	Am	Pm	Am	Pm	Am	Pm

Medication Log

Prescription	Am	Pm	Am	Pm	Am	Pm	Am	Pm

Medication Log

Prescription	Am	Pm	Am	Pm	Am	Pm	Am	Pm

Medication Log

Prescription	Am	Pm	Am	Pm	Am	Pm	Am	Pm

Medication Log

Prescription	Am	Pm	Am	Pm	Am	Pm	Am	Pm

Medication Log

Prescription	Am	Pm	Am	Pm	Am	Pm	Am	Pm

Medication Log

Prescription	Am	Pm	Am	Pm	Am	Pm	Am	Pm

Medication Log

Prescription	Am	Pm	Am	Pm	Am	Pm	Am	Pm

Medication Log

Prescription	Am	Pm	Am	Pm	Am	Pm	Am	Pm

Medication Log

Prescription	Am	Pm	Am	Pm	Am	Pm	Am	Pm

Medication Log

Prescription	Am	Pm	Am	Pm	Am	Pm	Am	Pm

Medication Log

Prescription	Am	Pm	Am	Pm	Am	Pm	Am	Pm

Medication Log

Prescription	Am	Pm	Am	Pm	Am	Pm	Am	Pm

Medication Log

Prescription	Am	Pm	Am	Pm	Am	Pm	Am	Pm

Symptom Tracker

This a great place to write down all of the symptoms that you are having. When you go to the doctors and he asks how you are feeling, you can tell him exactly what symptoms you had and how long you had them.

Symptom Tracker

	Nausea	Constipation	Diarrhea	Fatigue	Dizziness	Other
Sunday						
Monday						
Tuesday						
Wednesday						
Thursday						
Friday						
Saturday						

Symptom Tracker

	Nausea	Constipation	Diarrhea	Fatigue	Dizziness	Other
Sunday						
Monday						
Tuesday						
Wednesday						
Thursday						
Friday						
Saturday						

Symptom Tracker

	Nausea	Constipation	Diarrhea	Fatigue	Dizziness	Other
Sunday						
Monday						
Tuesday						
Wednesday						
Thursday						
Friday						
Saturday						

Symptom Tracker

	Nausea	Constipation	Diarrhea	Fatigue	Dizziness	Other
Sunday						
Monday						
Tuesday						
Wednesday						
Thursday						
Friday						
Saturday						

Symptom Tracker

	Nausea	Constipation	Diarrhea	Fatigue	Dizziness	Other
Sunday						
Monday						
Tuesday						
Wednesday						
Thursday						
Friday						
Saturday						

Symptom Tracker

	Nausea	Constipation	Diarrhea	Fatigue	Dizziness	Other
Sunday						
Monday						
Tuesday						
Wednesday						
Thursday						
Friday						
Saturday						

Symptom Tracker

	Nausea	Constipation	Diarrhea	Fatigue	Dizziness	Other
Sunday						
Monday						
Tuesday						
Wednesday						
Thursday						
Friday						
Saturday						

Symptom Tracker

	Nausea	Constipation	Diarrhea	Fatigue	Dizziness	Other
Sunday						
Monday						
Tuesday						
Wednesday						
Thursday						
Friday						
Saturday						

Symptom Tracker

	Nausea	Constipation	Diarrhea	Fatigue	Dizziness	Other
Sunday						
Monday						
Tuesday						
Wednesday						
Thursday						
Friday						
Saturday						

Symptom Tracker

	Nausea	Constipation	Diarrhea	Fatigue	Dizziness	Other
Sunday						
Monday						
Tuesday						
Wednesday						
Thursday						
Friday						
Saturday						

Symptom Tracker

	Nausea	Constipation	Diarrhea	Fatigue	Dizziness	Other
Sunday						
Monday						
Tuesday						
Wednesday						
Thursday						
Friday						
Saturday						

Symptom Tracker

	Nausea	Constipation	Diarrhea	Fatigue	Dizziness	Other
Sunday						
Monday						
Tuesday						
Wednesday						
Thursday						
Friday						
Saturday						

Symptom Tracker

	Nausea	Constipation	Diarrhea	Fatigue	Dizziness	Other
Sunday						
Monday						
Tuesday						
Wednesday						
Thursday						
Friday						
Saturday						

Symptom Tracker

	Nausea	Constipation	Diarrhea	Fatigue	Dizziness	Other
Sunday						
Monday						
Tuesday						
Wednesday						
Thursday						
Friday						
Saturday						

Symptom Tracker

	Nausea	Constipation	Diarrhea	Fatigue	Dizziness	Other
Sunday						
Monday						
Tuesday						
Wednesday						
Thursday						
Friday						
Saturday						

Symptom Tracker

	Nausea	Constipation	Diarrhea	Fatigue	Dizziness	Other
Sunday						
Monday						
Tuesday						
Wednesday						
Thursday						
Friday						
Saturday						

Symptom Tracker

	Nausea	Constipation	Diarrhea	Fatigue	Dizziness	Other
Sunday						
Monday						
Tuesday						
Wednesday						
Thursday						
Friday						
Saturday						

Symptom Tracker

	Nausea	Constipation	Diarrhea	Fatigue	Dizziness	Other
Sunday						
Monday						
Tuesday						
Wednesday						
Thursday						
Friday						
Saturday						

Symptom Tracker

	Nausea	Constipation	Diarrhea	Fatigue	Dizziness	Other
Sunday						
Monday						
Tuesday						
Wednesday						
Thursday						
Friday						
Saturday						

Symptom Tracker

	Nausea	Constipation	Diarrhea	Fatigue	Dizziness	Other
Sunday						
Monday						
Tuesday						
Wednesday						
Thursday						
Friday						
Saturday						

Symptom Tracker

	Nausea	Constipation	Diarrhea	Fatigue	Dizziness	Other
Sunday						
Monday						
Tuesday						
Wednesday						
Thursday						
Friday						
Saturday						

Symptom Tracker

	Nausea	Constipation	Diarrhea	Fatigue	Dizziness	Other
Sunday						
Monday						
Tuesday						
Wednesday						
Thursday						
Friday						
Saturday						

Symptom Tracker

	Nausea	Constipation	Diarrhea	Fatigue	Dizziness	Other
Sunday						
Monday						
Tuesday						
Wednesday						
Thursday						
Friday						
Saturday						

Symptom Tracker

	Nausea	Constipation	Diarrhea	Fatigue	Dizziness	Other
Sunday						
Monday						
Tuesday						
Wednesday						
Thursday						
Friday						
Saturday						

Symptom Tracker

	Nausea	Constipation	Diarrhea	Fatigue	Dizziness	Other
Sunday						
Monday						
Tuesday						
Wednesday						
Thursday						
Friday						
Saturday						

Symptom Tracker

	Nausea	Constipation	Diarrhea	Fatigue	Dizziness	Other
Sunday						
Monday						
Tuesday						
Wednesday						
Thursday						
Friday						
Saturday						

Symptom Tracker

	Nausea	Constipation	Diarrhea	Fatigue	Dizziness	Other
Sunday						
Monday						
Tuesday						
Wednesday						
Thursday						
Friday						
Saturday						

Symptom Tracker

	Nausea	Constipation	Diarrhea	Fatigue	Dizziness	Other
Sunday						
Monday						
Tuesday						
Wednesday						
Thursday						
Friday						
Saturday						

Symptom Tracker

	Nausea	Constipation	Diarrhea	Fatigue	Dizziness	Other
Sunday						
Monday						
Tuesday						
Wednesday						
Thursday						
Friday						
Saturday						

Symptom Tracker

	Nausea	Constipation	Diarrhea	Fatigue	Dizziness	Other
Sunday						
Monday						
Tuesday						
Wednesday						
Thursday						
Friday						
Saturday						

Symptom Tracker

	Nausea	Constipation	Diarrhea	Fatigue	Dizziness	Other
Sunday						
Monday						
Tuesday						
Wednesday						
Thursday						
Friday						
Saturday						

Symptom Tracker

	Nausea	Constipation	Diarrhea	Fatigue	Dizziness	Other
Sunday						
Monday						
Tuesday						
Wednesday						
Thursday						
Friday						
Saturday						

Symptom Tracker

	Nausea	Constipation	Diarrhea	Fatigue	Dizziness	Other
Sunday						
Monday						
Tuesday						
Wednesday						
Thursday						
Friday						
Saturday						

Symptom Tracker

	Nausea	Constipation	Diarrhea	Fatigue	Dizziness	Other
Sunday						
Monday						
Tuesday						
Wednesday						
Thursday						
Friday						
Saturday						

Food Journal

Use this to write down the foods that you eat during treatment. It always helps to know what you are eating for many reasons. You will know what makes you sick, gives you energy, smells funny, etc . . . And if you are like me, when chemo brain hits, you will want a place where everything is written down.

Weekly Food Journal

Week of_____ through_____

	Breakfast	Lunch	Dinner	Snacks
Sunday				
Monday				
Tuesday				
Wednesday				
Thursday				
Friday				
Saturday				

Weekly Food Journal

Week of_____ through_____

	Breakfast	Lunch	Dinner	Snacks
Sunday				
Monday				
Tuesday				
Wednesday				
Thursday				
Friday				
Saturday				

Weekly Food Journal

Week of_____ through_____

	Breakfast	Lunch	Dinner	Snacks
Sunday				
Monday				
Tuesday				
Wednesday				
Thursday				
Friday				
Saturday				

Weekly Food Journal

Week of_____ through_____

	Breakfast	Lunch	Dinner	Snacks
Sunday				
Monday				
Tuesday				
Wednesday				
Thursday				
Friday				
Saturday				

Weekly Food Journal

Week of_____ through_____

	Breakfast	Lunch	Dinner	Snacks
Sunday				
Monday				
Tuesday				
Wednesday				
Thursday				
Friday				
Saturday				

Weekly Food Journal

Week of_____ through_____

	Breakfast	Lunch	Dinner	Snacks
Sunday				
Monday				
Tuesday				
Wednesday				
Thursday				
Friday				
Saturday				

Weekly Food Journal

Week of_____ through_____

	Breakfast	Lunch	Dinner	Snacks
Sunday				
Monday				
Tuesday				
Wednesday				
Thursday				
Friday				
Saturday				

Weekly Food Journal

Week of_____ through_____

	Breakfast	Lunch	Dinner	Snacks
Sunday				
Monday				
Tuesday				
Wednesday				
Thursday				
Friday				
Saturday				

Weekly Food Journal

Week of_____ through_____

	Breakfast	Lunch	Dinner	Snacks
Sunday				
Monday				
Tuesday				
Wednesday				
Thursday				
Friday				
Saturday				

Weekly Food Journal

Week of_____ through_____

	Breakfast	Lunch	Dinner	Snacks
Sunday				
Monday				
Tuesday				
Wednesday				
Thursday				
Friday				
Saturday				

Weekly Food Journal

Week of_____ through_____

	Breakfast	Lunch	Dinner	Snacks
Sunday				
Monday				
Tuesday				
Wednesday				
Thursday				
Friday				
Saturday				

Weekly Food Journal

Week of_____ through_____

	Breakfast	Lunch	Dinner	Snacks
Sunday				
Monday				
Tuesday				
Wednesday				
Thursday				
Friday				
Saturday				

Weekly Food Journal

Week of_____ through_____

	Breakfast	Lunch	Dinner	Snacks
Sunday				
Monday				
Tuesday				
Wednesday				
Thursday				
Friday				
Saturday				

Weekly Food Journal

Week of_____ through_____

	Breakfast	Lunch	Dinner	Snacks
Sunday				
Monday				
Tuesday				
Wednesday				
Thursday				
Friday				
Saturday				

Weekly Food Journal

Week of_____ through_____

	Breakfast	Lunch	Dinner	Snacks
Sunday				
Monday				
Tuesday				
Wednesday				
Thursday				
Friday				
Saturday				

Weekly Food Journal

Week of_____ through_____

	Breakfast	Lunch	Dinner	Snacks
Sunday				
Monday				
Tuesday				
Wednesday				
Thursday				
Friday				
Saturday				

Weekly Food Journal

Week of_____ through_____

	Breakfast	Lunch	Dinner	Snacks
Sunday				
Monday				
Tuesday				
Wednesday				
Thursday				
Friday				
Saturday				

Weekly Food Journal

Week of_____ through_____

	Breakfast	Lunch	Dinner	Snacks
Sunday				
Monday				
Tuesday				
Wednesday				
Thursday				
Friday				
Saturday				

Weekly Food Journal

Week of_____ through_____

	Breakfast	Lunch	Dinner	Snacks
Sunday				
Monday				
Tuesday				
Wednesday				
Thursday				
Friday				
Saturday				

Weekly Food Journal

Week of_____ through_____

	Breakfast	Lunch	Dinner	Snacks
Sunday				
Monday				
Tuesday				
Wednesday				
Thursday				
Friday				
Saturday				

Weekly Food Journal

Week of_____ through_____

	Breakfast	Lunch	Dinner	Snacks
Sunday				
Monday				
Tuesday				
Wednesday				
Thursday				
Friday				
Saturday				

Weekly Food Journal

Week of_____ through_____

	Breakfast	Lunch	Dinner	Snacks
Sunday				
Monday				
Tuesday				
Wednesday				
Thursday				
Friday				
Saturday				

Weekly Food Journal

Week of_____ through_____

	Breakfast	Lunch	Dinner	Snacks
Sunday				
Monday				
Tuesday				
Wednesday				
Thursday				
Friday				
Saturday				

Weekly Food Journal

Week of_____ through_____

	Breakfast	Lunch	Dinner	Snacks
Sunday				
Monday				
Tuesday				
Wednesday				
Thursday				
Friday				
Saturday				

Weekly Food Journal

Week of_____ through_____

	Breakfast	Lunch	Dinner	Snacks
Sunday				
Monday				
Tuesday				
Wednesday				
Thursday				
Friday				
Saturday				

Weekly Food Journal

Week of_____ through_____

	Breakfast	Lunch	Dinner	Snacks
Sunday				
Monday				
Tuesday				
Wednesday				
Thursday				
Friday				
Saturday				

Weekly Calendar

Use this calendar for your doctor appointments, infusion appointments and as a record of visits from friends or family outings. It is good to have everything in one place. Not only for the time of your treatment but also to have so you can look back and see all that you have gone through and who was there to support you.

Week of: _____

Sunday	
Monday	
Tuesday	
Wednesday	
Thursday	
Friday	
Saturday	

Week of: _____

Sunday

Monday

Tuesday

Wednesday

Thursday

Friday

Saturday

Week of: _____

Sunday

Monday

Tuesday

Wednesday

Thursday

Friday

Saturday

Week of:

Sunday

Monday

Tuesday

Wednesday

Thursday

Friday

Saturday

Week of:_____

Sunday	
Monday	
Tuesday	
Wednesday	
Thursday	
Friday	
Saturday	

Week of: _____

Sunday

Monday

Tuesday

Wednesday

Thursday

Friday

Saturday

Week of:_____

Sunday

Monday

Tuesday

Wednesday

Thursday

Friday

Saturday

Week of: _____

Sunday

Monday

Tuesday

Wednesday

Thursday

Friday

Saturday

Week of:_____

Sunday

Monday

Tuesday

Wednesday

Thursday

Friday

Saturday

Week of: _____

Sunday	
Monday	
Tuesday	
Wednesday	
Thursday	
Friday	
Saturday	

Week of: _____

Sunday

Monday

Tuesday

Wednesday

Thursday

Friday

Saturday

Week of:_____

Sunday

Monday

Tuesday

Wednesday

Thursday

Friday

Saturday

Week of: _____

Sunday

Monday

Tuesday

Wednesday

Thursday

Friday

Saturday

Week of: _____

Sunday

Monday

Tuesday

Wednesday

Thursday

Friday

Saturday

Week of: _____

Sunday

Monday

Tuesday

Wednesday

Thursday

Friday

Saturday

Week of: _____

Sunday

Monday

Tuesday

Wednesday

Thursday

Friday

Saturday

Week of:_____

Sunday

Monday

Tuesday

Wednesday

Thursday

Friday

Saturday

Week of: _____

Sunday	
Monday	
Tuesday	
Wednesday	
Thursday	
Friday	
Saturday	

Week of:_____

Sunday
Monday
Tuesday
Wednesday
Thursday
Friday
Saturday

Week of:_____

Sunday

Monday

Tuesday

Wednesday

Thursday

Friday

Saturday

Week of: _____

Sunday

Monday

Tuesday

Wednesday

Thursday

Friday

Saturday

Week of:_____

Sunday	
Monday	
Tuesday	
Wednesday	
Thursday	
Friday	
Saturday	

Week of: _____

Sunday

Monday

Tuesday

Wednesday

Thursday

Friday

Saturday

Week of:

Sunday

Monday

Tuesday

Wednesday

Thursday

Friday

Saturday

Week of:_____

Sunday
Monday
Tuesday
Wednesday
Thursday
Friday
Saturday

Week of:_____

Sunday	
Monday	
Tuesday	
Wednesday	
Thursday	
Friday	
Saturday	

Disclaimer about this planner:

-This planner should not replace advice from a medical professional. Its design is for informational and support purposes only and is not a substitute for professional medical advice or treatment—for you or for anyone else.
-If you think you may have a medical emergency, call your physician or 911 immediately.
-The information in this planner should not be used for diagnosing or treating a health problem or disease.
-Always seek the advice of your physician or other qualified healthcare provider with any questions you may have regarding a medical condition.
-Reliance on any information provided by this planner is solely at your own risk.

Before Treatment

Try to relax while taking treatment. A few things that would be helpful to bring to your first treatment are: a book, laptop (for movies), headphones, or you might want to bring someone along. These things were great for me and helped keep my mind off of the drugs. If you are like me, it was hard for them to get an IV in, so drinking plenty of fluids before hand is a good idea. Wrap your arm in a blanket to keep your veins warm. I know it sounds funny, but it works.

During Treatment

You will have a window of time in between treatments when you are feeling somewhat yourself. Make sure that you do something fun for yourself and your family. Plan a day trip, go shopping, spend some alone time with your spouse. These things always helped me remember that this is only for a season. Write everything down. How you feel, side effects, things you liked, things you did not like. These things are very important to share with your doctor. They can adjust dosages and give you the correct ways to help you avoid having certain side effects.

After Treatment

Don't be alarmed if you don't bounce right back after treatment. Everyone is different and your body will eventually bounce back. Still try to take it easy and let people help you. The worst thing you could do is push yourself too hard. Take one day at a time and before you know it, your hair will be coming back, you will regain your sense of self, and your energy level will return to normal.

Notes

Notes

Notes

Notes

Notes

Notes

Notes

Notes

Notes

Notes

Notes

Notes

Notes

Notes

Notes

Notes

Notes

Notes

Notes

Notes